EXPOSI

8 Critical Takeaways for African Americans

EXPOSING DEMENTIA

---

8 Critical Takeaways for African American

C. Nathaniel Brown

EXPECTED END
ENTERTAINMENT

ATLANTA, GA

 Published by Expected End Entertainment. Address inquiries to: Expected End Entertainment P.O. Box 1751, Mableton, GA 30126.
ExpectedEndEntertainment@gmail.com
ISBN: 9781737146261

Printed in the United States of America

Contents

Dedication

This book is dedicated to my aunt and godmother Sheila Louise Brown.

Acknowledgements

Thank you to everyone who has embraced this journey to learn, sympathize and empathize with dementia patients, caregivers, and medical professionals in this space.

Thank you to everyone who has shared their stories for my documentary, *Remember Me: Dementia in the African American Community,* and this book. That list is extensive but each one of you is appreciated.

To Darlene, thank you for granting me the permission to share this portion of your story. You have contributed to a mission that will impact millions... for generations.

FOREWORD

Fayron Epps, PhD, RN,
Founder of Alter

Dementia is a term used to describe a group of symptoms affecting memory, thinking and social abilities in millions of individuals worldwide. It does not discriminate and is disproportionally impacting the African American community. Within the African American community, dementia presents unique cultural, social, and historical considerations that deserve special attention. Because of our history of social injustice and current issues with structural racism in America, African Americans have been made vulnerable, intentionally excluded, and thus disadvantaged. The very things that put us at a disadvantage and that make us vulnerable bring about disparities. Disparities are health differences that are avoidable, unnecessary, unfair, and unjust.

Exposing Dementia provides insights, direction, resources, and support for African Americans who want to enhance their knowledge. C. Nathaniel Brown offers culturally relevant insights about dementia and encourages African American families on this journey to "stay the course." He not only reflects on his personal story and the alarming statistics around dementia, but C. Nathaniel Brown also recognizes the critical need for the African American community to engage in research.

As a Black nurse scientist, I have devoted my career to reducing health disparities for underserved populations. My mission is to improve access to resources and awareness of dementia in Black and faith communities by conducting research and providing education. I work with Black churches to create culturally relevant dementia-related programs for their parishioners and community. When I am working with faith leaders, they often have shared with me they didn't know what dementia was. While conducting research with Black families living with dementia, I also heard their stories on how they felt the church – the one place they thought they could always count on – abandoned them. Involvement with clergy and congregants can also help persons living with dementia and their family members feel more comfortable and encouraged about their diagnosis. I have observed the positive impact of these tailored services on families who thought they couldn't attend worship services or include their family members living with dementia in the worship experience because of their circumstances.

Currently, there is no cure for dementia. However, there is a need to improve access to resources and awareness of dementia in the African American community. It is crucial that programs be developed to help those diagnosed with this condition and their families to understand the disease process and to live fully. I believe *Exposing Dementia* is responding to the needs of the African American community. C. Nathaniel Brown has crafted a resource and takeaways that are both informative and deeply empathetic to the experience of African Americans. *Exposing Dementia* is a culturally relevant resource that equips the African American community with knowledge on the medical, emotional, and practical dimensions of dementia. From the definition of dementia to the role of the Black church in this fight, this book provides invaluable insights for every African American family walking this path.

As African Americans, we need hope and education. We are such a hush-hush community, and that needs to end if we want better care and improved health outcomes. We cannot help each other if we do not take the time to learn about this disease and the reputable community resources and supportive services available for families. *Exposing Dementia* is an essential tool to break the silence about dementia in the African American community. African Americans can no longer be silent on this topic. Dementia can no longer be a "private family matter." I hope and pray that this book will help African American families speak up and feel more comfortable seeking support.

Faithfully,

Fayron Epps, PhD, RN, FGSA, FAAN
Founder, Alter™

Professor | Karen and Ronald Hermann Distinguished Chair in Caregiving
UT Health San Antonio School of Nursing

INTRODUCTION

Sometimes, you don't know what you don't know until you learn that you don't know it. That's exactly what happened to me when dementia stripped away my aunt's memories. When I saw her for the first time after she was diagnosed with dementia, my heart experienced a tremendous blow. In addition to being my aunt, Sheila Louise Brown is my godmother, who loved me and helped raise me like she birthed me. This day, she did not recognize me, or others who joined us for a dinner celebrating my mother. And her daughter, my cousin... she called her sister. The pain and the emotions overwhelmed me. I tried to hide it, but I couldn't release it. I still can't release it.

But when I returned from Baltimore to Atlanta, I tried to deal with it as I do most things... through my creative gift of writing, the same vehicle she encouraged me to use as a child. I wrote and produced a short film called, *That's My Brother*, a 7-minute film that shared a glimpse into what my aunt and cousin were dealing with. I played the son and an actor friend played my dad. I thought sharing this piece of life would ease the pain and emotions of what we were dealing with as a family. To the contrary, it revealed to me that a bigger mission, a bigger calling was at play.

When I released the film on YouTube and social media, it received a lot of love and positive feedback. But it also came with questions I couldn't answer. What type of dementia does your aunt have? Is it Alzheimer's disease? What stage is she in? What other symptoms is she experiencing? What treatment(s) is she on? The questions continued to roll in and I realized that I didn't know much at all about dementia.

From there, I did a deep dive to learn all that I could about dementia and what my aunt – and my uncle – were experiencing. It opened my eyes to the knowledge that I didn't know I needed, which had been hiding in plain sight. I learned what dementia was and many of its symptoms. I had only associated dementia with memory loss and disorientation. I learned the difference between dementia and Alzheimer's disease. I learned that there were more than 100 types of dementia. I learned about the challenges caregivers face. I learned about the disparities that impact the African American community. I learned about the dementia experts and caregiver advocates who are working extremely hard to help African Americans defeat dementia.

As a lifelong student with degrees and certificates across multiple disciplines, I was somewhat embarrassed that I knew so little about dementia. But I acknowledged a principle I adopted years ago… **"That which I learn, I will share!"** So, I decided to do what I do and produce another film, this time a documentary to help other African Americans learn about dementia and help loved ones care for those impacted.

As neuropsychologist Dr. Stephen Orey told me as I described what I would cover in my documentary, *Remember Me: Dementia in the African American Community*, "Be careful because you are going down a rabbit hole with no end." At that point, I was aware of it. I had already started planning a short documentary, maybe 30 minutes. At the time, I didn't know that I would be writing this book, but I knew the information needed to get in the hands of the people by any means necessary. The first version of the documentary was 3 hours long and I had so much more content to include and other interviews I still wanted to conduct. So I decided that I would cut the 3 hour documentary down to about an hour and 30 minutes and eventually do a 4-part series to get the rest of the information to the community.

That's my goal with this book... to share the information I acquired during the production of the documentary with the people who need it... the African American community which is disproportionately affected by dementia.

I know this book won't answer every question that dementia poses, but I believe it will help many to get a better understanding of what dementia is, how it impacts the African American community, some of the risk factors that we need to be aware of, and some tips to help us better care for ourselves and loved ones.

TAKEAWAY 1

WHAT IS DEMENTIA?

According to the National Institute of Aging, Dementia is the loss of cognitive functioning — thinking, remembering, and reasoning — to such an extent that it interferes with a person's daily life and activities. Some people with dementia cannot control their emotions, and their personalities may change. Dementia ranges in severity from the mildest stage, when it is just beginning to affect a person's functioning, to the most severe stage, when the person must depend completely on others for basic activities of daily living, such as feeding oneself.

Contrary to popular belief, dementia is not an inevitable consequence of getting older. But age is a risk factor, as we'll discuss in Chapter 2. Dementia is a specific medical condition characterized by cognitive decline that affects memory, thinking, and behavior. Each person who experiences dementia experiences it differently so some symptoms may present themselves in ways unique to that individual. But loss of memory is typically one of the first symptoms that presents itself.

Dementia is a global public health concern: The prevalence of dementia is increasing worldwide (55 million people), and it poses significant social and economic challenges. It is crucial to raise awareness and prioritize research efforts to develop effective treatments and improve care for individuals with dementia. Dementia is a growing public health issue worldwide. The number of people living with dementia is increasing, and the condition poses significant social and economic challenges. Raising awareness about dementia is vital to reduce stigma, improve access to healthcare services, and advocate for research funding to develop effective treatments and enhance the quality of care provided to individuals with dementia.

But it's impacting the African American and Latino communities harder than any other groups. According to the Alzheimer's Association, older African Americans are twice as likely as older white Americans to be diagnosed with Alzheimer's disease and other forms of dementia.

And with these statistics projected to get worse over the next 10-20 years, more needs to be done to reverse this trend. Experts say there are an additional 10 million people being diagnosed each year.

To reiterate, dementia is not a single disease: Dementia is an umbrella term that encompasses various diseases, the most common being Alzheimer's disease. Many people use dementia and Alzheimer's disease interchangeably. But they are not the same. Alzheimer's disease, which is caused by abnormal protein deposits in the brain that effects brain functioning, is a cause or a specific type of dementia. As one expert shared with me, you can have dementia without having Alzheimer's but you can't have Alzheimer's without having dementia.

As people watched my short film, *That's My Brother*, they began asking me questions that I couldn't answer. One of them was what type of dementia does my aunt have. I said, "What do you mean? It's dementia." That's when I began to hear some of the different causes of dementia such as Alzheimer's disease, Lewy body dementia, and vascular dementia. I had heard of Alzheimer's before but I never really understood what it, or dementia, entailed. My personal experience was limited to watching aging people deal with memory issues or hallucinations in the latter part of their lives and thinking, like most, this is just a part of getting older. The other causes or types of dementia I had never heard.

It caused me to dive in and find out more about the ones that were mentioned to me, leading me to discover that there were more than 100 types – or causes – of dementia. I was blown away by how little I knew about something that I now understand had impacted many in my family, including my grandmother, my biggest cheerleader. I learned that Alzheimer's accounted for 60-80% of all dementia cases. I also learned that Alzheimer's, vascular dementia and mixed dementia were most prevalent in the African American community.

Each type of dementia has its own underlying causes and unique characteristics. Some are identified by what is taking place in the brain, like the protein build up (Lewy body) or the reduced flow of oxygen to the brain (vascular dementia). Others are identified by where the changes take place in the brain (like frontotemporal dementia).

These more than 100 types of dementia cause the symptoms that we see in ourselves or our loved ones with dementia. Memory loss is usually the first symptom we notice, but it's not the only one. People with dementia may also experience difficulties with language, problem-solving, attention, and orientation. Changes in mood, personality, and behavior are also common. They may become irritated or agitated quicker than they used to. They may become more aggressive and even violent. People with dementia sometimes have problems finding the right words or following conversations. Problem-solving skills, attention span, and the ability to reason and make decisions may also be impaired. Additionally, individuals may struggle with orientation, finding it challenging to recognize familiar places or navigate their environment. There are other symptoms but those mentioned here are some of the more common ones.

Remember... each person's experience with dementia is unique. Proper diagnosis, ongoing medical care, and support are crucial for individuals with dementia and their caregivers. That's why it's crucial to consult medical professionals specializing in neurology, geriatrics, and dementia for accurate diagnosis, treatment, and management.

Below is a list of 100 types of dementia and a brief description of each. But there are more, and researchers are constantly discovering variations of existing ones.

1. **Alzheimer's Disease:** Alzheimer's is the most common type of dementia, characterized by the gradual deterioration of cognitive functions, memory loss, confusion, and impaired reasoning. It is caused by abnormal protein deposits, such as amyloid plaques and tau tangles, in the brain.
2. **Vascular Dementia:** Vascular dementia results from reduced blood flow to the brain due to strokes or other blood vessel-related issues. Symptoms include difficulties with memory, reasoning, and problem-solving, often occurring suddenly after a stroke.
3. **Lewy Body Dementia:** This type involves the buildup of abnormal protein deposits called Lewy bodies in the brain. It leads to fluctuations in cognitive abilities, visual hallucinations, Parkinson's-like motor symptoms, and significant variations in attention and alertness.
4. **Frontotemporal Dementia (FTD):** FTD is characterized by progressive damage to the frontal and temporal

lobes of the brain, leading to changes in personality, behavior, and language. There are different subtypes, including behavioral variant FTD and primary progressive aphasia.

5. **Parkinson's Disease Dementia:** Parkinson's disease can eventually lead to cognitive decline and dementia. Alongside motor symptoms like tremors and rigidity, individuals may experience memory problems, difficulty with multitasking, and changes in mood.
6. **Creutzfeldt-Jakob Disease (CJD):** CJD is a rare, rapidly progressing brain disorder caused by abnormal proteins called prions. It results in severe neurological symptoms, including rapid cognitive decline, muscle stiffness, and twitching.
7. **Huntington's Disease:** Huntington's is a hereditary disorder causing motor dysfunction, involuntary movements (chorea), and cognitive decline. Symptoms worsen over time and impact various aspects of a person's life.
8. **Mixed Dementia:** As the name suggests, mixed dementia involves a combination of different types of dementia, most commonly Alzheimer's disease and vascular dementia. This makes diagnosis and management more complex.
9. **Wernicke-Korsakoff Syndrome:** Often resulting from chronic alcohol abuse, this syndrome is characterized by severe memory impairment (Korsakoff's syndrome) and neurological symptoms due to a deficiency of thiamine (Vitamin B1).

10. **Normal Pressure Hydrocephalus (NPH):** NPH is caused by a buildup of cerebrospinal fluid in the brain's ventricles. Symptoms include difficulty walking, urinary incontinence, and cognitive impairment. Treating the fluid buildup can sometimes improve symptoms.
11. **Posterior Cortical Atrophy (PCA):** PCA is characterized by degeneration of the back part of the brain, leading to visual disturbances, difficulty recognizing objects, and challenges with reading and spatial awareness.
12. **Progressive Supranuclear Palsy (PSP):** PSP is a rare neurodegenerative disorder that affects movement and balance. Cognitive changes, including memory impairment and executive dysfunction, can also occur.
13. **Corticobasal Degeneration (CBD):** CBD is a rare neurodegenerative disorder characterized by movement problems, such as limb stiffness and jerky movements, as well as cognitive and language difficulties.
14. **Primary Progressive Aphasia (PPA):** PPA is a form of frontotemporal dementia that primarily affects language abilities. It leads to the gradual loss of speech and language skills while other cognitive functions may remain relatively intact.
15. **Posterior Cortical Atrophy (PCA):** PCA, also known as Benson's syndrome, primarily affects the back part of the brain responsible for processing visual information. It leads to difficulties with visual perception, spatial awareness, and recognition of objects and faces.
16. **Normal Pressure Hydrocephalus (NPH):** NPH is characterized by an accumulation of cerebrospinal fluid

in the brain's ventricles, causing gait problems, urinary incontinence, and cognitive impairment. Surgical intervention to drain the excess fluid can improve symptoms.

17. **Progressive Supranuclear Palsy (PSP):** PSP is a rare brain disorder that affects movement, causing balance problems, falls, and stiffness. Cognitive changes like memory loss and executive dysfunction can also occur.
18. **Subcortical Vascular Dementia:** This type of vascular dementia affects the deeper brain structures, leading to problems with movement, coordination, and cognition. It often results from small vessel disease and multiple small strokes.
19. **Traumatic Brain Injury (TBI)-Related Dementia:** Dementia can develop following a severe traumatic brain injury. Depending on the location and severity of the injury, cognitive impairment, memory problems, and personality changes may arise.
20. **AIDS-related Dementia:** Advanced stages of HIV infection can lead to cognitive impairment and dementia due to the virus affecting the brain's functioning. Symptoms include memory loss, confusion, and changes in behavior.
21. **Mixed Cortical and Subcortical Dementia:** This type involves a combination of cortical and subcortical brain damage, leading to a variety of symptoms, including cognitive decline, movement problems, and mood changes.
22. **Alcohol-Related Dementia:** Chronic alcohol abuse can lead to cognitive impairment and memory problems. It

may result from nutritional deficiencies, thiamine deficiency (Wernicke-Korsakoff syndrome), and direct brain damage.

23. **Chemotherapy-Induced Cognitive Impairment (CICI):** Some cancer patients undergoing chemotherapy may experience cognitive changes, often referred to as "chemo brain." This can involve memory problems, difficulty concentrating, and reduced cognitive processing speed.
24. **Metabolic Dementia:** Certain metabolic disorders, like Niemann-Pick disease and Gaucher's disease, can cause cognitive decline due to the accumulation of substances within brain cells.
25. **Down Syndrome-Related Dementia:** People with Down syndrome have an increased risk of developing Alzheimer's disease at a younger age due to the presence of an extra chromosome 21, which contains the gene associated with Alzheimer's.
26. **Dementia with Lewy Bodies (DLB):** DLB is similar to Parkinson's disease dementia, but the cognitive and motor symptoms appear simultaneously. Hallucinations, fluctuations in attention, and visual-spatial difficulties are common.
27. **Prion Diseases:** Prion diseases like Gerstmann-Sträussler-Scheinker (GSS) and Fatal Familial Insomnia (FFI) are extremely rare and involve abnormal proteins triggering progressive brain damage, leading to cognitive and motor impairments.
28. **Huntington's Disease-Like (HDL):** HDL refers to a group of conditions that resemble Huntington's disease in

terms of movement problems and cognitive decline but lack the genetic mutation associated with Huntington's. These disorders are often collectively referred to as "Huntington's disease phenocopies."

29. **CADASIL (Cerebral Autosomal Dominant Arteriopathy with Subcortical Infarcts and Leukoencephalopathy):** CADASIL is a hereditary condition caused by mutations in a specific gene, resulting in blood vessel abnormalities within the brain. It leads to recurrent strokes, cognitive impairment, and mood disturbances.
30. **Frontotemporal Lobar Degeneration (FTLD):** FTLD is an umbrella term encompassing multiple types of frontotemporal dementia. It includes behavioral variant FTD (bvFTD) characterized by personality and behavioral changes, as well as primary progressive aphasia (PPA), affecting language abilities.
31. **Late-Onset Tay-Sachs Disease:** Tay-Sachs disease typically presents in infancy, but a rarer late-onset variant can manifest in adulthood. It leads to progressive cognitive and motor decline due to the accumulation of certain lipids in the brain.
32. **Lafora Disease:** Lafora disease is a rare genetic disorder leading to epilepsy and cognitive decline. It's characterized by the accumulation of abnormal proteins called Lafora bodies within cells.
33. **FTD with Motor Neuron Disease (MND):** This is a subtype of frontotemporal dementia that includes symptoms of motor neuron disease (similar to amyotrophic lateral sclerosis or ALS), leading to both cognitive and motor impairments.

34. **Primary Age-Related Tauopathy (PART):** PART is characterized by the presence of tau protein deposits in the brain, similar to Alzheimer's disease, but to a lesser extent. It can lead to cognitive changes, particularly in memory.
35. **Dementia Pugilistica:** Also known as chronic traumatic encephalopathy (CTE), this type of dementia is associated with repetitive head trauma, often seen in athletes participating in contact sports. Symptoms include mood changes, memory problems, and cognitive decline.
36. **Mitochondrial Dementia:** Mitochondrial disorders, which affect the energy-producing structures within cells, can lead to cognitive impairment due to reduced energy supply to brain cells.
37. **LATE (Limbic-Predominant Age-Related TDP-43 Encephalopathy):** LATE is a recently recognized type of dementia characterized by abnormal accumulations of TDP-43 protein. It primarily affects memory and is more common in older adults.
38. **Neuronal Ceroid Lipofuscinosis (NCL):** Also known as Batten disease, NCL refers to a group of rare genetic disorders causing progressive brain degeneration in children. It leads to seizures, motor decline, and cognitive impairment.
39. **Prion-Like Dementias:** These are a group of disorders that share characteristics with prion diseases, involving the misfolding and aggregation of proteins. Disorders like frontotemporal dementias with tau mutations and

certain types of Parkinson's disease are considered prion-like.

40. **Multisystem Atrophy (MSA):** MSA is a rare neurodegenerative disorder with symptoms resembling Parkinson's disease and autonomic dysfunction. Cognitive impairment can also occur, but it's often less prominent than the motor and autonomic symptoms.
41. **Neuronal Intranuclear Inclusion Disease (NIID):** NIID is a rare genetic disorder characterized by abnormal protein accumulations within the nucleus of nerve cells. It leads to a variety of neurological symptoms, including cognitive decline and movement problems.
42. **Alexander Disease:** This rare genetic disorder affects astrocytes, a type of brain cell. It results in a range of neurological symptoms, including cognitive impairment, seizures, and movement difficulties.
43. **Retinal Vasculopathy with Cerebral Leukoencephalopathy and Systemic Manifestations (RVCL-S):** RVCL-S is a rare condition affecting both the brain and the eyes. It causes cognitive decline, strokes, and vision problems due to abnormalities in blood vessel walls.
44. **Senescent Cell-Associated Brain Dysfunction (SABD):** SABD refers to age-related cognitive decline associated with the accumulation of senescent (aging) cells in the brain. These cells release inflammatory molecules that contribute to cognitive impairment.
45. **FTD with Amyotrophic Lateral Sclerosis (ALS):** This subtype of frontotemporal dementia involves symptoms of both frontotemporal dementia and ALS, a

progressive motor neuron disease. It leads to cognitive and motor impairments.

46. **Dementia associated with Autoimmune Encephalitis:** Certain autoimmune conditions can cause inflammation in the brain, leading to cognitive and behavioral changes. Anti-NMDA receptor encephalitis and Hashimoto's encephalopathy are examples.
47. **Neimann-Pick Disease Type C:** A rare genetic disorder, Niemann-Pick Type C leads to the accumulation of lipids within cells. It results in neurological symptoms, including cognitive decline, movement problems, and seizures.
48. **Malnutrition-Related Dementia:** Severe malnutrition, particularly deficiencies in vitamins and minerals, can lead to cognitive impairment. Conditions like pellagra (niacin deficiency) and beriberi (thiamine deficiency) are examples.
49. **Dementia in Cerebral Autosomal Recessive Arteriopathy with Subcortical Infarcts and Leukoencephalopathy (CARASIL):** CARASIL is a genetic disorder that affects blood vessels in the brain, leading to cognitive decline, movement difficulties, and psychiatric symptoms.
50. **Cholinergic Overdrive Dementia:** Cholinergic overdrive refers to an excessive release of acetylcholine, a neurotransmitter. This can lead to cognitive symptoms, often seen in individuals with Lewy body dementia.
51. **Binswanger's Disease:** Also known as subcortical vascular dementia, Binswanger's disease is caused by damage to the small blood vessels deep within the

brain. It leads to cognitive decline, mood changes, and difficulty walking.

52. **Amyloid Angiopathy-Related Dementia:** Amyloid angiopathy involves the buildup of amyloid protein in blood vessels of the brain. This can lead to cognitive impairment and an increased risk of cerebral hemorrhages.
53. **Limbic Encephalitis:** Limbic encephalitis is an autoimmune disorder that primarily affects the limbic system, leading to memory problems, seizures, mood changes, and hallucinations.
54. **Progressive Myoclonic Epilepsy-Related Dementia:** Certain forms of progressive myoclonic epilepsy can lead to cognitive decline, movement difficulties, and myoclonus (involuntary muscle jerks).
55. **Chronic Traumatic Encephalopathy (CTE):** CTE is associated with repetitive head trauma, often seen in athletes and individuals with a history of concussions. It causes cognitive, mood, and behavioral changes.
56. **Late-Onset Frontotemporal Dementia:** This form of frontotemporal dementia occurs later in life and shares similar symptoms with early-onset FTD, including personality changes, language difficulties, and impaired judgment.
57. **Dementia in Multiple Sclerosis (MS):** In some cases of multiple sclerosis, cognitive impairment can develop. It can involve problems with memory, attention, and processing speed due to lesions and inflammation in the brain.

58. **Focal Cortical Dysplasia-Related Dementia:** Focal cortical dysplasia is a brain malformation that can lead to epilepsy and cognitive decline. It involves abnormal development of brain tissue in specific areas.
59. **CADASIL Variant:** This is a variant of CADASIL (Cerebral Autosomal Dominant Arteriopathy with Subcortical Infarcts and Leukoencephalopathy) that presents with similar symptoms but may involve distinct genetic mutations.
60. **Primary Progressive Multiple Sclerosis (PPMS):** PPMS is a type of multiple sclerosis characterized by the gradual accumulation of disability. Cognitive changes, such as memory problems and difficulties with concentration, can also occur.
61. **Dementia associated with Chronic Kidney Disease:** Chronic kidney disease can impact brain function due to factors like electrolyte imbalances, toxins buildup, and vascular issues, leading to cognitive impairment.
62. **Dementia associated with Chronic Obstructive Pulmonary Disease (COPD):** Severe cases of COPD, a lung disease, can result in oxygen deprivation to the brain, leading to cognitive changes and memory problems.
63. **Dementia associated with Congestive Heart Failure (CHF):** Congestive heart failure can affect blood flow to the brain, leading to cognitive impairment, confusion, and difficulty with attention and memory.
64. **Prion-Like Tauopathy:** This type of dementia involves the spread of abnormal tau protein in a prion-like manner, similar to Creutzfeldt-Jakob disease. It's

associated with cognitive decline and memory problems.

65. **Subacute Sclerosing Panencephalitis (SSPE):** SSPE is a rare disorder caused by a persistent measles virus infection. It leads to progressive brain inflammation, cognitive decline, and seizures.
66. **Dementia associated with HIV:** Advanced HIV infection can lead to cognitive impairment, often referred to as HIV-associated neurocognitive disorders (HAND). It involves memory problems, decreased attention, and executive dysfunction.
67. **Lymphomatosis Cerebri:** This rare condition involves the infiltration of lymphoma cells within the brain's white matter, leading to cognitive decline, seizures, and neurological symptoms.
68. **Leukoencephalopathy with Brainstem and Spinal Cord Involvement and Lactate Elevation (LBSL):** LBSL is a genetic disorder characterized by white matter abnormalities in the brain. It can lead to motor and cognitive impairments, as well as movement difficulties.
69. **Dementia associated with Hypothyroidism:** Severe hypothyroidism can lead to cognitive changes, memory problems, and difficulties with concentration due to a reduced level of thyroid hormone.
70. **MELAS Syndrome (Mitochondrial Encephalomyopathy, Lactic Acidosis, and Stroke-like Episodes):** MELAS is a mitochondrial disorder that can cause cognitive impairment, seizures, and stroke-like episodes due to energy production issues within cells.

71. **CADASIL Variant:** A variant of CADASIL (Cerebral Autosomal Dominant Arteriopathy with Subcortical Infarcts and Leukoencephalopathy) that involves different genetic mutations, leading to similar symptoms like cognitive decline and stroke-like episodes.
72. **Glutaric Aciduria Type 1:** A rare metabolic disorder that can lead to brain damage due to the accumulation of certain acids. It results in movement problems, cognitive decline, and seizures.
73. **Hyper IgM Syndrome-Associated Dementia:** Hyper IgM syndrome is an immune system disorder that, in certain cases, can cause cognitive impairment due to inflammation and damage to the brain.
74. **Charcot-Marie-Tooth Disease Type 1A (CMT1A):** A hereditary neurological disorder affecting peripheral nerves, CMT1A can lead to muscle weakness and atrophy, as well as cognitive impairment in some cases.
75. **Binswanger's Disease Variant:** A variant of Binswanger's disease involving distinct characteristics, such as different patterns of white matter lesions, leading to cognitive impairment, mood changes, and difficulty walking.
76. **MERRF Syndrome (Myoclonic Epilepsy with Ragged Red Fibers):** MERRF is a mitochondrial disorder characterized by myoclonic seizures, muscle weakness, and cognitive decline due to energy production deficits in cells.
77. **Hypoparathyroidism-Related Dementia:** Hypoparathyroidism, a condition involving low levels of

parathyroid hormone, can lead to cognitive impairment, memory problems, and mood changes.

78. **Hereditary Diffuse Leukoencephalopathy with Spheroids (HDLS):** A rare genetic disorder causing damage to the brain's white matter, HDLS leads to cognitive decline, movement problems, and mood changes.
79. **Rett Syndrome:** A genetic disorder primarily affecting girls, Rett syndrome leads to severe cognitive and physical impairments, loss of purposeful hand skills, and repetitive movements.
80. **SCA17 (Spinocerebellar Ataxia Type 17):** A type of hereditary ataxia, SCA17 can lead to both movement difficulties and cognitive decline, along with other symptoms like involuntary eye movements.
81. **CADASIL Variant:** Another variant of CADASIL (Cerebral Autosomal Dominant Arteriopathy with Subcortical Infarcts and Leukoencephalopathy) that involves distinct genetic mutations, leading to cognitive decline, mood changes, and stroke-like symptoms.
82. **Hepatic Encephalopathy:** Hepatic encephalopathy is caused by liver dysfunction, leading to a buildup of toxins in the blood that can affect brain function. It results in cognitive impairment, confusion, and altered consciousness.
83. **Dementia associated with Hypercalcemia:** Abnormally high levels of calcium in the blood can lead to cognitive changes, confusion, and memory problems.
84. **Kearns-Sayre Syndrome:** A mitochondrial disorder that often manifests in childhood, Kearns-Sayre syndrome

leads to muscle weakness, vision problems, and cognitive decline.

85. **Progressive Encephalopathy with Edema, Hypsarrhythmia, and Optic Atrophy (PEHO) Syndrome:** PEHO syndrome is a rare genetic disorder causing severe brain dysfunction, leading to cognitive and motor impairment, seizures, and visual problems.
86. **Hypoglycemia-Related Dementia:** Severe episodes of low blood sugar levels can lead to cognitive impairment, confusion, and difficulty with attention and memory.
87. **Dementia associated with Chronic Liver Disease:** Chronic liver disease, such as cirrhosis, can lead to cognitive decline, memory problems, and confusion due to toxic substances not being efficiently cleared from the blood.
88. **Wernicke's Encephalopathy:** Caused by a deficiency of thiamine (Vitamin B1), Wernicke's encephalopathy leads to cognitive impairment, confusion, and difficulties with coordination and movement.
89. **Acute Disseminated Encephalomyelitis (ADEM):** ADEM is an autoimmune disorder that often follows viral infections. It leads to inflammation in the brain and spinal cord, resulting in cognitive decline, seizures, and movement problems.
90. **Neuroacanthocytosis Syndromes:** This group of rare genetic disorders, including Chorea-acanthocytosis and McLeod syndrome, causes movement problems, cognitive decline, and the presence of abnormal red blood cells (acanthocytes).

91. **Marchiafava-Bignami Disease:** This rare disorder is associated with alcohol abuse and leads to damage of the corpus callosum, resulting in cognitive impairment, seizures, and motor dysfunction.
92. **Dementia associated with Hyperthyroidism:** Excessively high levels of thyroid hormone can lead to cognitive changes, irritability, and difficulties with concentration.
93. **Sporadic Creutzfeldt-Jakob Disease (sCJD):** This is the most common form of Creutzfeldt-Jakob disease, a rare prion disorder causing rapidly progressive cognitive decline, muscle stiffness, and twitching.
94. **Adult Polyglucosan Body Disease:** A rare genetic disorder leading to the accumulation of complex sugars in cells, adult polyglucosan body disease causes cognitive impairment, muscle weakness, and bladder problems.
95. **Autosomal Recessive Cerebellar Ataxia:** This group of disorders involves genetic mutations that lead to cerebellar degeneration, resulting in both movement difficulties and cognitive decline.
96. **Aicardi-Goutières Syndrome:** A rare genetic disorder causing inflammation in the brain, Aicardi-Goutières syndrome leads to cognitive regression, seizures, and movement problems.
97. **Dementia associated with Wilson's Disease:** Wilson's disease involves the buildup of copper in the body, affecting the brain and liver. It can lead to cognitive impairment, movement difficulties, and psychiatric symptoms.

98. **Progressive Nonfluent Aphasia (PNFA):** PNFA is a subtype of frontotemporal dementia primarily affecting language abilities, resulting in difficulties with speech production and syntax while other cognitive functions may remain relatively intact.
99. **Fucosidosis:** A rare lysosmal storage disorder, fucosidosis leads to progressive cognitive and motor impairment due to accumulation of certain substances within cells.
100. **Adult-Onset Metachromatic Leukodystrophy (MLD):** A rare genetic disorder involving the loss of myelin, the protective coating of nerve cells, adult-onset MLD leads to cognitive decline, movement problems, and psychiatric symptoms.

TAKEAWAY 2

DEMENTIA RISK FACTORS

Several risk factors contribute to the higher incidence and diagnosis of dementia among African Americans. These risk factors can be categorized into various domains, including genetic and biological factors, lifestyle and environmental factors, and social determinants of health. Here are some key risk factors:

Genetic factors: Certain genetic variations and susceptibility genes can increase the risk of developing dementia. While the exact genetic mechanisms underlying dementia in African Americans are still being studied, there is evidence to suggest that genetic factors may contribute to the higher prevalence of dementia in this population.

Cardiovascular health: Cardiovascular risk factors, such as hypertension, diabetes, obesity, and high cholesterol, are more prevalent among African Americans. These conditions can contribute to the development of vascular dementia and increase the risk of other types of dementia, including Alzheimer's disease.

Educational attainment: Lower levels of educational attainment, which can be influenced by socioeconomic factors and systemic inequities, have been associated with an increased risk of dementia. Educational disparities among African Americans may contribute to the higher incidence of dementia in this population.

Socioeconomic factors: Socioeconomic factors, such as income level, occupation, and access to resources, can impact health outcomes, including the risk of dementia. African Americans may experience socioeconomic disparities, including lower income levels, limited access to healthcare, and higher rates of poverty, which can increase the risk of dementia.

Health disparities and healthcare access: African Americans often face disparities in healthcare access, quality of care, and health outcomes. Limited access to healthcare services, delays in diagnosis, and inadequate management of chronic conditions may contribute to an increased risk of dementia among African Americans.

Psychosocial factors: Psychosocial factors, such as stress, depression, and social isolation, can influence the risk of dementia. African Americans may face unique psychosocial stressors, including racial discrimination, socioeconomic challenges, and cultural factors, which can contribute to increased dementia risk. Psychosocial factors play a significant role in influencing the risk of dementia, and African Americans may face unique psychosocial stressors that can contribute to increased risk. Here's a closer look at how these factors impact dementia risk within the African American community:

Racial discrimination: African Americans often face experiences of racial discrimination and systemic racism, which can lead to chronic stress and psychological distress. Chronic exposure to racial discrimination has been linked to negative health outcomes, including an increased risk of cognitive decline and dementia.

Socioeconomic challenges: African Americans are more likely to experience socioeconomic challenges, including lower income levels, higher rates of poverty, and limited access to resources.

Socioeconomic disadvantage can lead to chronic stress, limited opportunities for healthcare, and increased risk of dementia.

Cultural factors: Cultural factors, such as cultural beliefs, values, and caregiving norms, can influence dementia risk. African Americans may have cultural practices that impact health behaviors, help-seeking attitudes, and caregiving approaches. Understanding and addressing cultural factors are important for providing culturally sensitive dementia care and support.

Social isolation: Social isolation and limited social support networks can contribute to increased dementia risk. African Americans may face social isolation due to various factors, such as living in segregated neighborhoods, limited access to community resources, and the impact of historical and ongoing societal inequities.

Depression and mental health: Depression and other mental health conditions are more prevalent among African Americans, and these conditions are associated with an increased risk of dementia. The experience of racial discrimination, socioeconomic challenges, and other psychosocial stressors can contribute to the development of mental health disorders, further impacting dementia risk.

It is important to recognize and address these psychosocial stressors to mitigate the impact on dementia risk within the African American community. Promoting mental health awareness, providing culturally competent mental health support, addressing systemic racism, and improving socioeconomic opportunities are crucial steps in reducing the psychosocial burden and dementia risk among African

Americans. Additionally, fostering supportive and inclusive communities that promote social connections and combat social isolation can help mitigate the negative impact of psychosocial factors on dementia risk.

It is important to note that these risk factors are complex and interact with each other. Additionally, individual experiences and variations within the African American population can influence the impact of these risk factors on dementia risk. Addressing these risk factors requires a comprehensive approach that includes promoting cardiovascular health, improving educational opportunities, reducing health disparities, increasing access to healthcare, and addressing social determinants of health.

TAKEAWAY 3

EARLY DIAGNOSES and TREATMENT

As the journey through the intricate landscape of dementia unfolds, there is a critical crossroad that every individual and their loved ones must traverse—early diagnosis. Imagine standing at the threshold of a path that could profoundly influence the course of this challenging journey. This chapter aims to illuminate the significance of embarking on this path early, highlighting the benefits of early diagnosis and the essential steps to take for effective treatment.

The Unseen Power of Early Detection

In the realm of dementia, time is both a precious ally and an elusive adversary. Early diagnosis empowers individuals and their caregivers with the knowledge needed to make informed decisions, paving the way for proactive interventions that can enhance quality of life and potentially slow the progression of the condition. By identifying the specific type of dementia and its underlying causes, healthcare professionals can tailor treatment plans to address the unique needs and challenges each individual faces.

But why is early diagnosis so pivotal? At its core, dementia involves complex neurological changes that often begin subtly, gradually eroding cognitive functions, memory, and daily living abilities. Detecting these changes early can open windows of opportunity to implement strategies that mitigate their impact. Early intervention can help preserve cognitive function, optimize medication management, and offer psychological support to both individuals and their families.

But unfortunately, African Americans are least likely to seek medical attention at the onset of most of the symptoms. When we do, we are often ignored, misdiagnosed, or told to wait until things get worse. African Americans rarely have access to the best information, resources or treatments when we do seek help.

Navigating the Treatment Terrain

Once an individual receives an early diagnosis of dementia, the next phase involves charting a thoughtful course of treatment. While dementia itself is not curable, its symptoms and progression can be managed through a comprehensive approach that addresses physical, cognitive, emotional, and social aspects. Here are crucial steps to consider:

1. Collaborate with Healthcare Professionals

Forming a strong partnership with healthcare professionals specializing in dementia care is essential. Neurologists, geriatricians, psychiatrists, and dementia specialists bring their expertise to the table, tailoring treatment plans to the individual's needs and preferences.

Collaboration with healthcare professionals who specialize in dementia care is crucial following an early diagnosis. These specialists bring a wealth of knowledge and experience to guide individuals and their families through the complexities of dementia. Neurologists, geriatricians, psychiatrists, and dementia specialists work together to develop a holistic treatment plan tailored to the individual's needs.

During the early stages of dementia, healthcare professionals conduct thorough assessments to determine the type of dementia, its underlying causes, and the individual's overall health status. This information serves as the foundation for creating a personalized care plan that addresses specific challenges and goals.

2. Implement Cognitive Interventions

Cognitive interventions encompass a spectrum of activities designed to engage and stimulate the mind. These interventions can help slow cognitive decline, improve memory, and enhance overall cognitive function. Activities might include brain training exercises, puzzles, memory games, and engagement in hobbies or creative endeavors.

Cognitive interventions are strategies designed to preserve and enhance cognitive function. Engaging in mentally stimulating activities can help slow cognitive decline and maintain brain health. Brain training exercises, puzzles, memory games, and even learning new skills or languages can keep the mind active and agile.

These interventions not only benefit the individual with dementia but also provide opportunities for meaningful interactions with caregivers and loved ones. Additionally, they contribute to a sense of accomplishment and satisfaction, promoting a positive emotional state.

3. Medication Management

In many cases, medication can help manage specific symptoms of dementia, such as memory loss, mood changes, and sleep disturbances. Early diagnosis allows healthcare providers to prescribe medications that are most appropriate for the individual's type of dementia and overall health.

While medications cannot reverse dementia, they can help manage specific symptoms, improving overall quality of life. Early diagnosis allows healthcare providers to prescribe medications that are most appropriate for the type of dementia and the individual's medical history.

For example, medications may be prescribed to alleviate memory problems, manage mood changes, and address sleep disturbances. Healthcare professionals closely monitor the individual's response to medication and make necessary adjustments to ensure optimal effectiveness.

4. Lifestyle Modifications

Healthy lifestyle choices play a pivotal role in managing dementia. Encouraging regular physical exercise, a balanced diet rich in brain-boosting nutrients, and proper sleep hygiene can have a positive impact on cognitive function.

Healthy lifestyle choices play a significant role in managing the progression of dementia. Regular physical exercise has been shown to support brain health by promoting blood flow, reducing inflammation, and enhancing neuroplasticity—the brain's ability to adapt and reorganize.

A balanced diet rich in nutrients like antioxidants, omega-3 fatty acids, and B vitamins can also support cognitive function. Adequate sleep is essential for memory consolidation and overall brain health. By promoting these lifestyle modifications, individuals can positively impact their cognitive well-being.

5. Psychological and Emotional Support

Dementia affects not only cognitive function but also emotional well-being. Early diagnosis provides the opportunity to establish psychological support mechanisms, such as counseling or therapy, which can help individuals and families navigate the emotional challenges that may arise.

Early diagnosis opens the door to psychological and emotional support, addressing the emotional challenges that often accompany dementia. Counseling, therapy, and support groups can provide individuals and their families with tools to cope with grief, anxiety, and other emotional stressors.

These support mechanisms help individuals develop coping strategies, manage feelings of loss, and promote emotional resilience. By addressing emotional well-being alongside cognitive function, early diagnosis contributes to a comprehensive approach to dementia care.

6. Caregiver Education and Support

Early diagnosis not only benefits the individual with dementia but also empowers caregivers with knowledge about the condition. Caregiver support groups, educational resources, and respite care services can ease the caregiving journey and prevent burnout.

Early diagnosis doesn't just benefit the person with dementia—it extends to caregivers as well. Caregivers play a vital role in the journey, providing physical and emotional support. Education about the condition, its progression, and caregiving strategies equips caregivers with the knowledge and skills to provide effective care.

Support groups offer caregivers a platform to share experiences, exchange advice, and find comfort in the understanding of others facing similar challenges. Respite care services also give caregivers opportunities for temporary relief, reducing the risk of burnout and promoting their own well-being.

The Path Forward

The decision to seek an early diagnosis of dementia is an empowering step toward gaining control over an uncertain future. It is a choice that sets the stage for informed decision-making, personalized interventions, and a higher quality of life. I hope this chapter serves as a guiding light, illuminating the significance of early diagnosis and underscoring the transformative impact it can have on the lives of those affected by dementia. The journey is challenging, but with the right information and support, it is a journey that can be navigated with resilience and grace.

In the words of Dr. Orey:

"We gotta take care of us!"

The importance of early diagnosis in dementia cannot be overstated. Each step in the treatment process, from collaborating with healthcare professionals to implementing cognitive interventions and providing emotional support, contributes to a comprehensive and holistic approach to care.

Early diagnosis empowers individuals and their families to make informed decisions, optimize treatment strategies, and maintain the best possible quality of life throughout the dementia journey. By embracing these steps, individuals affected by dementia can navigate their path with greater resilience, hope, and a sense of purpose.

TAKEAWAY 4

DISPARITIES IN DEMENTIA

As stated in Chapter 1, dementia is a growing crisis worldwide with more than 55 million people already diagnosed and that number growing by more than 10 million annually.

Dementia affects people from all racial and ethnic backgrounds. While there is limited research specifically focused on the impact of dementia on African Americans, studies suggest that we face unique challenges and disparities in dementia care. Here are some statistics that shed light on the impact of dementia on African Americans:

- ***Higher prevalence:*** According to estimates from the Alzheimer's Association, African Americans are about twice as likely as non-Hispanic whites to develop Alzheimer's disease or other dementias. However, the exact reasons for this disparity are still being investigated.
- ***Earlier onset:*** Research suggests that African Americans tend to develop dementia at an earlier age compared to non-Hispanic whites. This earlier onset can have significant implications for the affected individuals and their families, including prolonged caregiving responsibilities and financial burdens.
- ***Underdiagnosis and misdiagnosis:*** African Americans may be less likely to receive a timely and accurate diagnosis of dementia. Various factors, including limited access to healthcare, lower rates of health insurance coverage, and cultural beliefs and stigma surrounding mental health, can contribute to underdiagnosis and misdiagnosis.

- ***Lower awareness and knowledge:*** Studies indicate that African Americans may have lower levels of awareness and knowledge about dementia compared to other racial and ethnic groups. This lack of awareness can lead to delayed help-seeking behaviors and limited access to available resources and support services.

While there is limited specific research on the awareness and knowledge of dementia among African Americans, several studies have explored the general trends and factors influencing dementia awareness in diverse populations. These studies provide insights into the lower levels of awareness and knowledge about dementia within the African American community. Here are some key findings:

The Aging, Demographics, and Memory Study (ADAMS): The ADAMS, conducted by the National Institute on Aging, investigated dementia prevalence and awareness among different racial and ethnic groups in the United States. The study found that compared to non-Hispanic whites, African Americans had lower levels of dementia awareness and were less likely to report memory problems to their healthcare providers.

The REasons for Geographic and Racial Differences in Stroke (REGARDS) study: The REGARDS study examined racial and geographic disparities in health outcomes, including cognitive decline. The research indicated that African Americans had lower knowledge about dementia symptoms and were less likely to identify memory loss as a potential sign of dementia compared to whites.

The Alzheimer's Association's "Generation Alzheimer's" study: This nationwide survey explored awareness, attitudes, and caregiving experiences related to Alzheimer's disease. The study found that African Americans had lower levels of knowledge about Alzheimer's disease compared to other racial and ethnic groups. They were less likely to recognize the warning signs of dementia and had lower confidence in their ability to recognize those signs.

Community-based studies: Studies conducted within African American communities have highlighted the lack of awareness and knowledge about dementia. These studies have shown that many African Americans have limited familiarity with the term "dementia" and may use alternative terms or concepts to describe cognitive decline, such as "nervous breakdown" or "senility."

These studies suggest that lower levels of dementia awareness among African Americans may stem from various factors, including limited access to health education, cultural beliefs, language barriers, and historical mistrust of the healthcare system. Lack of awareness can lead to delayed help-seeking behaviors, as individuals may not recognize the symptoms of dementia or understand the importance of seeking timely medical evaluation.

Addressing the awareness gap requires community-based educational initiatives that specifically target African American populations. Culturally tailored educational programs, public awareness campaigns, and partnerships with community organizations can help increase knowledge about dementia, its symptoms, available resources, and the importance of early diagnosis and treatment. Empowering community leaders, healthcare providers, and caregivers to disseminate accurate information and engage in open dialogue is vital in improving dementia awareness within the African American community.

That's why I HAD to do something! I know this book won't reach every African American. I know the documentary won't be seen by every African American. But I am confident that together they will reach millions of African Americans across the country and others of the African diaspora to introduce them to the knowledge I've acquired. This is my *"it takes a village"* message that somewhere along the line has fallen by the wayside. Additionally, I hope both projects inspire and motivate others outside of the African diaspora who genuinely care about the world and its people to help us make these life-changing and life-sustaining changes. But it starts with us.

We have to identify those among us who can carry the torch through advocacy, financial support, the arts, medicine, the church, and every other area where we can reach African Americans. That's the only way we'll be able to reverse the growing numbers of disparities that affect us. The harvest is plentiful but the laborers are few.

- **Caregiving challenges:** African American families often play a crucial role in providing care for individuals with dementia. Due to socioeconomic factors and limited access to support services, African American caregivers may face additional challenges, such as higher caregiving burden, financial strain, and limited respite care opportunities.

- **Disparities in healthcare access and quality:** African Americans may face disparities in accessing quality healthcare services, including dementia diagnosis, treatment, and management. These disparities can be influenced by factors such as socioeconomic status, geographic location, and implicit biases within the healthcare system. Disparities in healthcare for African Americans refer to the unequal access to quality healthcare services, differences in health outcomes, and variations in the quality of care received compared to other racial and ethnic groups. These disparities can be influenced by various factors, including socioeconomic status, implicit biases within the healthcare system, and structural inequities. Here are some key aspects of healthcare disparities affecting African Americans:
- **Access to healthcare:** African Americans often face barriers to accessing healthcare services, including limited health insurance coverage, financial constraints, and inadequate proximity to healthcare facilities. Lack of access can result in delayed or forgone medical care, including preventive services and timely diagnosis of conditions like dementia.
- **Diagnosis and treatment disparities:** Studies have shown disparities in the diagnosis and treatment of diseases among African Americans. This can include delays in the diagnosis of conditions like dementia, resulting in missed opportunities for early interventions and management. African Americans may also receive

different treatment options or lower quality care compared to other racial and ethnic groups.

- **Implicit biases and cultural competence:** Implicit biases, both conscious and unconscious, can influence healthcare providers' attitudes and treatment decisions. African Americans may experience prejudice, stereotyping, or inadequate cultural understanding from healthcare professionals, leading to suboptimal care. Culturally competent care, which acknowledges and addresses the unique needs and experiences of African Americans, is crucial for equitable healthcare delivery.
- **Health literacy and communication:** Limited health literacy among African Americans can hinder their ability to understand healthcare information, navigate the healthcare system, and actively participate in decision-making. Language barriers, low educational attainment, and disparities in health information access can contribute to these challenges. Effective communication strategies, such as plain language, visual aids, and interpreter services, are essential to bridge this gap and promote better health outcomes.
- **Chronic disease management:** African Americans experience higher rates of chronic diseases, such as diabetes, hypertension, and cardiovascular disease, which are risk factors for dementia. Disparities in disease management and control contribute to the overall health burden. Access to regular healthcare, medication adherence, and lifestyle interventions are critical for managing these conditions and potentially reducing the risk of dementia.

Addressing healthcare disparities requires a comprehensive approach that tackles both individual and systemic factors. Strategies include improving healthcare access, increasing diversity in the healthcare workforce, enhancing cultural competency training for healthcare providers, promoting health literacy and patient empowerment, and implementing policies that address socioeconomic determinants of health. By addressing these disparities, it is possible to improve the overall health outcomes and well-being of African Americans, including in the context of dementia care.

Addressing these disparities and improving dementia care for African Americans requires a multi-faceted approach. This includes raising awareness about dementia within the African American community, promoting culturally sensitive healthcare practices, increasing access to quality healthcare services, and supporting caregivers through targeted resources and support networks. Additionally, further research is needed to better understand the underlying causes of these disparities and develop tailored interventions to address them effectively.

STATISTICS/DATA:

- African Americans are approximately two times more likely to develop Alzheimer's disease compared to non-Hispanic whites.
- According to estimates, African Americans represent about 13.4% of the U.S. population aged 65 and older but account for approximately 33% of individuals living with Alzheimer's disease.

- African Americans are more likely to be diagnosed with Alzheimer's disease in the later stages, which may indicate delays in seeking medical help or accessing appropriate diagnostic services.
- Compared to non-Hispanic whites, African Americans with dementia are more likely to have vascular dementia, a type of dementia caused by reduced blood flow to the brain.
- Higher rates of cardiovascular risk factors, such as hypertension and diabetes, contribute to the increased risk of dementia among African Americans.
- Socioeconomic factors play a role in dementia risk. African Americans with lower educational attainment and income levels may face a higher risk of developing dementia.
- Caregiving for African Americans with dementia is often provided by family members, with higher levels of informal caregiving observed within the community.
- Access to dementia care and support services may be limited for African Americans due to healthcare disparities and underutilization of available resources.
- Studies have shown that African Americans may have lower levels of awareness and knowledge about dementia, leading to delayed diagnosis and treatment.
- Cultural factors, such as beliefs and attitudes toward dementia and caregiving, influence the experiences and outcomes of African Americans living with dementia.

TAKEAWAY 5

HISTORICAL MISTRUST of the MEDICAL COMMUNITY

The distrust of the medical field and the United States government among African Americans has deep historical roots, with various incidents contributing to this mistrust. Here are five examples that highlight reasons behind this distrust:

Tuskegee Syphilis Study: The Tuskegee Syphilis Study, conducted by the U.S. Public Health Service from 1932 to 1972, is one of the most notorious examples of medical mistreatment. African American men with syphilis were deceived and denied proper treatment, even after the discovery of penicillin as an effective cure. The study violated ethical standards and led to long-lasting mistrust of the medical establishment.

Henrietta Lacks and HeLa cells: Henrietta Lacks, an African American woman, had her cells taken without her consent in 1951 for medical research. These cells, known as HeLa cells, became crucial for scientific advancements but were used without the knowledge or consent of Lacks or her family. This case raised concerns about ethical practices, informed consent, and the exploitation of marginalized communities.

Forced sterilizations: Forced sterilizations were performed on African American women, often without their informed consent, as part of eugenics programs in the United States. These programs aimed to control population growth among marginalized groups and disproportionately targeted African Americans. Such practices have contributed to a legacy of mistrust and fear of reproductive healthcare services.

Experiments on enslaved individuals: During the era of slavery, enslaved individuals were subjected to medical experiments without their consent or consideration for their well-being. These experiments, which involved procedures, surgeries, and medical testing, were conducted for the benefit of medical knowledge and the advancement of medical practices. This history of exploitation has engendered a deep sense of mistrust.

Racial disparities in healthcare: Persistent racial disparities in healthcare outcomes, including higher rates of chronic diseases, maternal mortality, and limited access to quality healthcare, contribute to the mistrust of the medical field. African Americans have historically experienced inequities in healthcare delivery and have often received substandard care, reinforcing a perception of systemic bias and neglect.

It is important to note that these examples represent only a fraction of the historical mistreatment and systemic inequities experienced by African Americans. Recognizing and addressing these past injustices is crucial to rebuilding trust and working towards equitable healthcare practices that respect the rights and well-being of all individuals, regardless of their race or ethnicity.

The mistreatment and systemic inequities experienced by African Americans throughout history are numerous and pervasive. Here are some additional examples that highlight the depth of these injustices:

- Slavery and Jim Crow era: The institution of slavery and the subsequent Jim Crow era were characterized by systemic racism, segregation, and pervasive discrimination against African Americans. These periods enforced social, economic, and political disparities, denying African Americans basic human rights, education, economic opportunities, and access to healthcare.
- Lynchings and racial violence: African Americans faced rampant lynchings and racial violence throughout history. Lynching, often carried out with impunity, was a horrific tool of racial terrorism, instilling fear and subjugation within African American communities. The legacy of racial violence

contributes to the ongoing trauma and mistrust experienced by African Americans.

- Segregated healthcare: During the era of segregation, African Americans faced segregated healthcare facilities, limited access to medical services, and disparities in the quality of care provided. Separate and unequal medical systems perpetuated health disparities, leading to poorer health outcomes for African Americans.
- Redlining and housing discrimination: Redlining, a discriminatory practice prevalent during the mid-20th century, systematically denied African Americans access to housing and perpetuated residential segregation. Limited access to quality housing often translated into inadequate living conditions, reduced access to resources, and diminished overall well-being, including healthcare access.
- Disproportionate incarceration and criminal justice system biases: African Americans have faced disproportionate rates of incarceration, often as a result of systemic biases within the criminal justice system. The over-policing of African American communities, racial profiling, and disparities in sentencing contribute to the perpetuation of systemic inequities and erode trust in the justice system.
- Education disparities: African Americans have long faced disparities in education, including unequal access to quality schools, resources, and opportunities. Segregated schooling, underfunding of schools serving predominantly African American communities, and racial disparities in educational outcomes contribute to the cycle of systemic inequity.

These examples represent only a fraction of the historical mistreatment and systemic inequities experienced by African Americans. It is important to recognize this legacy of oppression and systemic racism as it continues to impact various aspects of African

American lives, including healthcare, education, economic opportunities, and overall well-being. Addressing these historical injustices and working towards meaningful systemic change is essential for achieving racial equity and justice.

TAKEAWAY 6

RESEARCH and CLINICAL TRIALS

Dementia research is advancing rapidly, offering hope for improved understanding, treatments, and ultimately, a cure. Staying informed about the latest developments and supporting organizations dedicated to dementia research is crucial for progress in the field. Continued research is essential to develop effective interventions, enhance care practices, and ultimately find a way to prevent or cure dementia.

Dr. Antoine Trammell is a researcher and dementia expert who diligently attempts to enlist more African Americans into dementia research and clinical trials. In *Remember Me*, he talks about some of the challenges he and other researchers face because of the years of mistreatment by the United States government and the medical community. But he also emphasizes the importance of making the necessary changes to improve our lifestyle. He said that new advances are being made but without increased African American participation, some of the new medications and treatments might not be as effective in our community. But he has hope.

In 2023, the U.S. Food and Drug Administration converted Leqembi (lecanemab-irmb), indicated to treat adult patients with Alzheimer's disease, to traditional approval following a determination that a confirmatory trial verified clinical benefit. Leqembi is the first amyloid beta-directed antibody to be converted from an accelerated approval to a traditional approval for the treatment of Alzheimer's disease. The drug works by reducing amyloid plaques that form in the brain, a defining pathophysiological feature of the disease.

According to Teresa Buracchio, acting director of the Office of Neuroscience in the FDA's Center for Drug Evaluation and Research, Leqembi "is the first verification that a drug targeting the underlying disease process of Alzheimer's disease has shown clinical benefit in this devastating disease."

This is exciting news for Alzheimer's patients, caregivers, and researchers alike. It means progress is being made and there is hope that one day there will be a cure for dementia.

There are hundreds of studies and trials currently taking place around the world. But many are lacking African American participation, some intentionally excluding African Americans and others can't break the barrier that the mistrust created. That's why researchers like Dr. Trammell, Dr. Stephanie Johnson, and others are pushing for more African American researchers and more targeted recruitment by African Americans of African Americans.

Dr. Trammell believes the Leqembi approval will ultimately lead to other research and treatment, which is why it's imperative that more African Americans participate.

I interviewed Jackie Collins-Riddick who was recently diagnosed with Alzheimer's disease. She said she is participating in dementia trials and studies with the hopes that it will prevent future generations from experiencing what she is experiencing. Ms. Collins-Riddick told me that it takes courage and selflessness to step outside of your comfort zone for something that will benefit you and your family.

Researchers know there is still a steep hill to climb. Many are learning about Henrietta Lacks and her family's story after Oprah Winfrey produced a film based on the injustice done to her. In 2019, Lou Gossett Jr. portrayed a musician with Alzheimer's disease in a film called The Cuban. With more awareness of dementia, more Black researchers, and the new advancements in treatment, I am hopeful that the African American participation will rise.

TAKEAWAY 7

CAREGIVING

A caregiver is a person who tends to the needs or concerns of a person with short- or long-term limitations due to illness, injury or disability. That could be a family member or someone hired to assist, such as a nurse.

Within the African American community, many family members become caregivers of loved ones with dementia. There are several reasons for this including: lack of trust with outsiders caring for loved ones; financial limitations; keeping illnesses secret; and denial of the severity of the illness until it's necessary to seek outside support.

According to Healthline.com, home care for an older adult with dementia may run anywhere from $25-$40/hour, which translates to about $4,000-$6,400/month for full-time care (based on a 40-hour workweek). However, the cost can be higher in some states or areas with a higher cost of living.

The Alzheimer's Association says some of the common care cost for Alzheimer's patients include:

- Ongoing medical treatment for Alzheimer's-related symptoms, diagnosis and follow-up visits.
- Treatment or medical equipment for other medical conditions.
- Safety-related expenses, such as home safety modifications or safety services for a person who wanders.
- Prescription drugs.
- Personal care supplies.
- Adult day care services.
- In-home care services.

- Full-time residential care services.

The Alzheimer's Association also said many people don't consider long-term care services which include home- and community-based services, assisted living and nursing home care.

- **Home care**: A paid non-medical home health aide is $28.64 per hour and $1,145 per week (assuming 40 hours of care per week).
- **Adult day services**: $83 per day.
- **Assisted living facilities**: $4,774 per month or $57,289 per year.
- **Private room in a nursing home**: $315 per day or $115,007 per year.
- **Semi-private room in a nursing home**: $276 per day or $100,679 per year.

As you can see, dementia can have far-reaching effects on families' finances, especially in low income communities where the risk factors are magnified and the dementia numbers are skyrocketing. And many families are forced to take on the full-time role of caregiver because there are not many other options.

Dementia also has impact on other areas for caregivers, and communities. As a community, we need to understand the challenges faced by caregivers and provide them with support. Unfortunately, we don't often know what our family members or neighbors are dealing with. The more we discuss these topics, the less taboo dementia and caregiving are. We must combat the stigma that is associated with health issues, especially with dementia and cognitive challenges in general. Caregivers are crucial in this discussion. Caregivers, especially unpaid family caregivers, need support, and caregivers need to ask for help.

Family members, friends, and caregivers often bear a significant burden in terms of emotional, physical, and financial challenges. Recognizing and addressing the needs of caregivers is crucial to ensure their well-being and their ability to provide effective support.

One of the areas I discovered during interviews for *Remember Me* was the increasing depression rates among dementia patients, which I understood. But what I couldn't imagine prior to the documentary was how prevalent depression and suicide are among caregivers. Caregivers expressed how they were overwhelmed, depressed and in need of care, too. Compassion fatigue is real. That's why the depression rate and the suicide rates are skyrocketing.

My writing client and good friend Sharise Nance is a licensed therapist and compassion fatigue expert. In the documentary, she pulled from several of her books to speak about the importance of recognizing fatigue while caring for others. She called compassion fatigue the common cold for those in the helping profession, which includes caregivers. She stressed how oftentimes, we try to handle everything on our own without getting the support and therapy we need.

Several people in the documentary, including Sharise, Senior 911 owner Sonja Gunter, and support group facilitator Dawnita Brown, introduced me to the term respite. Respite is a short period of rest or relief from something usually difficult.

I got a chance to spend some time at Tender Living Care Adult Day Center in Snellville, GA. It's a dementia day center where owner Jennifer Harris and her team focuses on keeping each client present with exercises, brain games, and various art activities such as painting and dancing. The center is open during from 8 a.m. to 5 p.m., which allows family caregivers to work, shop, or do other activities they wouldn't be able to do without some type of respite service.

Sonja's business provides in-home respite services, in which dementia-trained nurses sit with dementia patients while family members run errands or take self-care time.

According to the National Institute of Health, 85% of caregivers do not take advantage of respite services.

In addition to having that respite, most experts say it's imperative to have a support system around the caregiver and for the caregiver to participate in support groups with others who can relate to what they are dealing with.

Here are 10 tips to help caregivers who are taking care of individuals with dementia:

- ***Educate yourself:*** Learn as much as you can about dementia, its symptoms, and progression. Understanding the condition can help you anticipate and address challenges effectively.
- ***Seek support:*** Don't hesitate to reach out for support. Join caregiver support groups or seek counseling to connect with others who are going through similar experiences and gain valuable insights and advice.

- ***Establish a routine:*** Creating a consistent daily routine can provide structure and familiarity for the person with dementia. Routines help reduce confusion and anxiety and can make caregiving tasks more manageable.
- ***Simplify tasks:*** Break down tasks into smaller, manageable steps to help the person with dementia complete them. Provide clear and simple instructions, and be patient and supportive throughout the process.
- ***Practice effective communication:*** Use clear and concise language, speak slowly, and maintain a calm tone. Use visual cues, gestures, and touch to enhance communication. Listen attentively and validate the person's feelings.
- ***Ensure safety:*** Make the environment safe by removing hazards, securing doors and windows, and installing grab bars or handrails as needed. Consider utilizing monitoring devices or alarms to enhance safety.
- ***Take care of yourself:*** Remember to prioritize your own physical, emotional, and mental well-being. Take breaks, engage in self-care activities, and seek respite care to prevent burnout and maintain your own health.
- ***Maintain social connections:*** Stay connected with friends, family, and support networks. Social interactions and maintaining relationships outside of caregiving provide emotional support and prevent isolation.
- ***Seek professional help:*** Don't hesitate to consult healthcare professionals, such as doctors, nurses, or therapists, to address specific concerns or seek

guidance on managing challenging behaviors or symptoms.

- ***Celebrate moments of joy:*** Find joy in the small moments and celebrate successes, however small they may be. Engage in activities that the person with dementia enjoys, such as listening to music, going for walks, or engaging in hobbies, to promote a positive and fulfilling experience.

Remember, caregiving can be challenging, but with support, education, and self-care, you can provide the best possible care for your loved one with dementia while taking care of yourself. At the end of this book, I have included a resource list for caregivers to assist you on this journey.

TAKEAWAY 8

CHANGING the PERCEPTION of DEMENTIA

Depending on which study you read, it's suggested that it takes between 18 and 254 days to form a habit. Well, my question is how long will it take to change the perception of dementia in the African American community?

As stated earlier, dementia has been growing at staggering numbers and has found its way into the daily global healthcare discussions. But discussing dementia in the African American community is still considered somewhat taboo, even though it's been around and impacting Black people for hundreds of years.

Dr. Orey explained how through the years the Black community labeled symptoms of dementia under various names and titles including senility and mental breakdowns. But most often, the derogatory term of "crazy" has been thrown about when people in the community experience mental and physical symptoms that were outside of their normal personality.

As a result of such negativity, people suffering depression, memory loss, and thinking challenges, often conceal what they are experiencing from others, including family members. Rather than share what they are experiencing to get the help they need, many simply keep their challenges to themselves, suffering in silence. One of my cousins, who is just 46, has suffered three strokes. Several family members *and* friends have told her she doesn't need to walk with a cane and ridicule her when she experiences brain fog or memory loss. So, to avoid those encounters, she often chooses to deal with her challenges in silence.

In other cases, extended family members who feared the public shame or ridicule from outside their home, perpetuated the idea of "What happens in this house, stays in this house."

That thought process hasn't helped the African American community. In fact, it has hurt it. It's imperative that we change many of the practices that have plagued the African American community through the years. We must begin to discuss the issues that are ripping through the community including gun violence, sex trafficking, healthcare disparities, depression, suicide... and yes, dementia.

The bible says in Hosea 4:6 - "My people are destroyed from lack of knowledge." Sometimes, we don't know that our lack of knowledge is what is killing us. Other times, our willingly rejecting knowledge exacerbates the problems in the African American community.

Martin Luther King Jr. once said, "The function of education is to teach one to think intensively and to think critically. Intelligence plus character – that is the goal of true education." In another speech, he said, "...complete education gives one not only power of concentration, but worthy objectives upon which to concentrate."

I did a private screening of *Remember Me* for my mother, and two of my cousins. All three were aware of what I was trying to accomplish with the documentary. I interviewed my mother and my cousin, Darlene, for the project. My other cousin, Keir, and I had brief conversations via Facebook after I discovered her strokes put her at greater risk for dementia. They had all seen the trailer prior to this get together.

But after watching the documentary, they were blown away by the amount of information they learn about dementia, despite having multiple family members currently suffering from it and several who died with some form of dementia.

It was another "Ah-ha" moment for me as well. The first was when I began researching after *That's My Brother*. Just like then, I could see beyond the immediate thoughts and emotions of this new information and new experience. We began having an intimate and emotional conversation that started with what we can do for ourselves, then shifted to what we could do to help others.

Changing the perception of something that has been so entrenched in a community isn't easy. Like the Chinese proverb says, "A journey of a thousand miles begins with a single step." For me, I knew I had to take a step when I was overcome with emotion behind my aunt's memory loss. But I thought it was personal. After I discovered that it was much more than that, much bigger than that, I was thrust into being one of the people charged with helping to change the perception of dementia in my community.

One of my personal mission statements that I've used as a topic during speaking engagements is: "To help people dream bigger, live their dreams and impact their world." Your world is not necessarily continents or countries. Your world could be in your home, on your job, at your gym, or at the parent-teachers association. For *Remember Me*, I started at home with my family. And my family received the messages and I believe the call to action to make a difference in their own lives and then *their world*.

So, what can we need to do to change the perception of dementia in the African American community? I thought about the 12-Steps of Alcoholics Anonymous and Narcotics Anonymous (which are similar to other addiction processes). Honesty. Faith. Surrender. Soul-Searching. Integrity.

Acceptance. Humility. Willingness. Forgiveness. Maintenance. Making Contact. Service. We need to take a similar approach to changing perception around dementia because for years we've perfected bad habits and behaviors that I believe have contributed to the disparities. If we are going to improve as a community, we need a concerted effort and plan to overcome the years of self-sabotage. Here are five areas that I've discovered during my research and interviews for *Remember Me* that encompass many of the 12-step components and that I believe will make a significant difference:

1. **Pray** – Prayer changes things. There is no way we can change hundreds of year of abuse, disparities, mistrust, and behavior on our own. We need God today more than ever before. Step 2 of AA and NA, is faith, which says to accept that there is a higher power that can help change your perspective, hold you accountable and make a difference in your journey. I'm a believer in Jesus Christ and I have experienced the types of miracles we need on *this* journey. So I will continue to pray for all those impacted by dementia.
2. **Take Care of Yourself** – In addition to being a caregiver, my friend Linda Michelle Trainer is a flight attendant of 30 years. She cared for her late mother who suffered from Alzheimer's and is now caring for her husband, who has Alzheimer's. In *Remember Me*, she uses the analogy of placing your oxygen mask on first before trying to assist someone else. This means to make sure you get checked out if you find

something is off in your mental or physical condition because early prevention and treatment are critical to maintaining a good quality of life. You're no good to others if you're not good yourself. If you are a caregiver, take advantage of respite, support groups, and self-care programs. If you need help, don't be afraid to ask for it.

3. **Learn More About Dementia** – Thanks to research, clinical trials and more people sharing their stories, there is more information about dementia becoming available every day. We have access to much of this material to increase our knowledge about general information such as definitions and statistics to specific information such as medications for different types/causes of dementia. With the internet so accessible, there is no excuse for being unaware. Commit to learning more about dementia so the conversations become easier.
4. **Share Information** – You don't need to be a doctor, nurse or therapist to share knowledge you acquire. That's the purpose of the documentary and this book... to share what I've discovered, hoping it will reach some people that otherwise would have never received it. When you stumble across a great article discussing dementia, forward it to your family and friends. Tell them about a movie that has dementia as a theme. Share a book for caregivers with someone you know who could use it. Remember, impact your world! Tell your

stories or help others tell their stories. And if you need help, reach out to us.

5. **Support Dementia Patients and Caregivers** – Dr. Fayron Epps is founder of Alter, a program that helps to create dementia friendly atmospheres in churches. Since Black churches have always been the cornerstone of the African American experience in the United States, Dr. Epps works to funnel information through pastors and faith institutions. There are also other organizations helping dementia patients and caregivers in need. You may want to start a support group, contribute to a fundraiser or volunteer at a memory care day center. Ask how you can support, then show up. I love the saying I heard in sports… "The best ability is availability".

CONCLUSION

CALL to ACTION

Do something! Anything! Help us fight dementia by showing up for those impacted and by supporting caregivers because dementia is fighting the African American community, and sadly it's winning. The statistics show that and we're not talking about it enough, we're not doing enough about it, and by the time many of us are affected personally, it's too late.

I've decided to do my part, whatever that is or whatever it will be because I want all of us to be better, do better and live better for as long as God sees fit. *Thanks My Brother* was a start, and I thought it was just for me but so many others received from it. *Remember Me* has already received a few film festival awards and I pray it reaches the millions of people who need to see it. I pray this book does the same.

I often think about a famous quote from rapper Tupac Shakur, in which he says:

"I'm not saying I'm gonna change the world, but I guarantee that I will spark the brain that will change the world."

I'm not saying I'm going to defeat dementia, but I'm hoping that my contributions make a difference. I hope that something you read will ignite a spark in you that will strengthen you to continue your fight. I believe this book and the documentary are divine assignments from God. I am called to be obedient and to do my part, whatever that is. I don't have a medical degree. I'm not a nurse. I'm not a dementia specialist. I am a storyteller with purpose. And like Tupac, I believe the sparks that are *Exposing*

Dementia: 8 Critical Takeaways for African Americans, and *Remember Me: Dementia in the African American Community*, will spark something in someone to do something remarkable in this fight against dementia.

Maybe for you it's sharing your dementia story, or providing respite for a caregiver so they can continue to serve their loved one. There are no small roles to this puzzle. The smallest piece is just as significant as the largest one. You can't complete the puzzle without all the pieces in their proper places. You are important. Do something.

Virtual Dementia Tour

You may need to do some research, take classes, or attend support groups to get the necessary information to find out where you need to be and what you need to do.

I participated in a virtual dementia tour, which builds sensitivity and awareness for individuals caring for those with dementia by temporarily altering participants' physical and sensory abilities. I won't go into details because I don't want to ruin the experience for those who may participate in one later. But I highly recommend it because it helps you to understand many things that those without dementia take for granted. It also allows you to empathize with dementia patients. It was certainly life-changing for me.

Here are some of my takeaways from that experience:

1. I found myself doing things that my uncle and aunt do that I didn't understand why before the tour.

2. I understand better the frustration and agitation over the simple tasks that we take for granted.
3. The concept of time left as soon as I entered the room.
4. The anxiety I experienced was overwhelming.
5. My compassion level increased with the experience.
6. I immediately felt the charge to do more to help those in the fight against dementia.

I'm grateful for that opportunity, but my heart was aching even more for my family members and the people I met and interviewed for the documentary. I began recommending people to participate in the tour. Again, it's a small thing but it made a significant impact in my life. I believe the more people who participate in the tour and similar dementia awareness trainings, the more will be engaged in making a difference for our loved ones and for generations to come.

To you who are battling any form of dementia, my prayers are with you. Keep the faith and continue to cherish every moment you can with your family and friends. Steve and Danita Jefferson, a couple featured in the documentary shared something with me. Steve is just 50 years old and has been battling dementia for roughly 10 years. He has lost a lot of his memory. But Danita has made it a point to create new memories every day. On the good days that Steve remembers their wedding some 19 years ago, they stay in that moment. When he doesn't, they cherish the trips they go on to create new ones.

Stay in the moment. Enjoy what you can and who you can for as long as you can. Don't take a second for granted. I know that you won't.

That also should apply to family and friends of dementia patients. In the documentary, my cousin said she wished she could have one more conversation with her mother where she knew who she was and they could just talked about anything, maybe share a common memory.

Our responsibility now is to cherish every moment and implement things that will prolong the time we have with our loved ones and teach the younger generations to take better care of themselves so they can live a long, prosperous life dementia free. That starts with each of us taking action to make a difference in our families, in our communities, and in whatever sphere of influence we have.

To caregivers... I hope you found comfort in these pages and that you, too, realize you are not alone. You are loved and you are appreciated, even if the person you care for doesn't know it or can't express it. In your caring, care for yourself.

Ms. Collins-Riddick shared these words in the documentary:

"Love yourself enough to pay attention to you because you are the most important person you know."

During the editing process of the documentary, I probably listened to that clip 1,000 times. And each time it resonates with me. Caregiving takes a measure of selflessness. And that's admirable, especially when it comes to our loved ones. But you are no good to them if you are not good yourself. So, take care of yourself. Talk to other caregivers, join support groups, talk to a therapist, take advantage of respite services, and get refueled for the work you do. I celebrate you. You are valued. You are loved.

At the end of this book, I have compiled a list of resources for dementia patients and a list for caregivers. I'm sure others can take advantage of several organizations that are on the front line of the battle, including Second Wind Dreams, the virtual dementia tour group.

Let's work together to understand dementia better, help eradicate the disparities, become more compassionate as a group, rid the stigma of dementia in our community, and support those in need – dementia patients, caregivers, advocates, researchers, etc.

I believe in us. We are the strongest, most resilient people on earth. We have overcome so many obstacles. Dementia will be the next one.

TRIBUTE to my AUNT/my GODMOTHER

Sheila Louise Brown

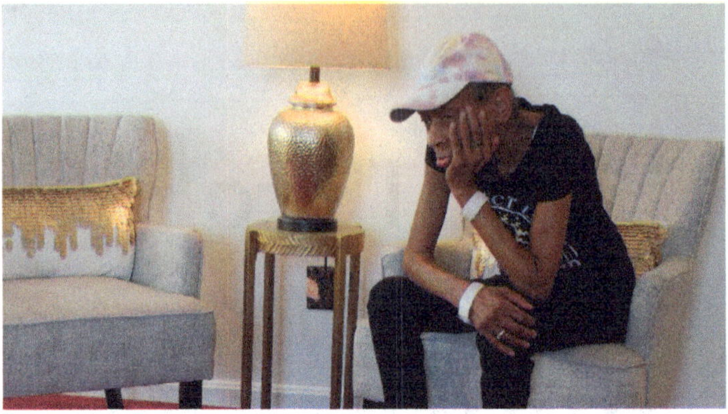

That's my aunt, my godmother Sheila Louise Brown. From before I could remember, she was like a second mother to me raising me along with her own daughter just like she birthed me. That's why her daughter and I have always been closer than cousins; we are brother and sister.

My aunt taught me things like cooking certain food, being respectful to adults, how to read, how to do multiplication and division, and how to throw a right hook to defend myself from the bullies who used to chase me home.

I miss the stories she'd share every time she saw me. They'd be the same ones... reciting the first poem I ever wrote...

"I don't like cabbage.

I don't like rice.

I like you

'cus you are nice."

I remember it today because of all the times she recited it. She wrote me 2 poems in response to my poem... "My Food Gets Winks" and "My Food Still Gets Winks" that she talked about every time I saw her.

To: Chuck

I Can't Write Poetry but My Food Gets Winks

By Sheila L. Brown ©1992

Many have said my poetry stinks
but I'm not hurt because my food gets winks
It was first brought to my attention while in class
I had to write a poem or I couldn't pass
Upon completion of my task, I felt very good
My poem would sound terrific… I knew it would
That day at school I sat up strong and tall
My class was an advanced one and very small
I sat on the edge of my seat for my name to be called
Most of the other students' poetry I didn't understand
The average of the poems were about the inhumanity of man
When my name was called, I sprang to my feet
I moved so fast I almost knocked over my seat
I read my poem with glitter and glee
At least I was finished and my mind was free
The criticism (by classmates) was heartless and cruel
But critical estimates and discussion were a part of the class rule
When they finished I felt like a dunce
I wanted to cry and leave the room at once

I knew I was not Maya Angelou
And found out it was true
So, Chuck my poetry may stink
But to many my food still get winks

She'd share the story of how she taught me to punch a bully in the solar plexus and how I defended my female cousins from an older, bigger neighborhood guy, throwing him onto a car.

Even if she didn't get all the details right or embellished some for the sake of making them more interesting, you could count on at least one, two or three stories that connected you to her.

She was always proud of me, and she made sure I knew it. She made sure I knew that she loved me and encouraged me to tell those I loved what they meant to me. She credited herself with teaching me how to talk to girls when I was a skinny, shy teenager.

My aunt was a teacher who loved to impart wisdom on all who came around her, especially little children. She was adamant about starting the learning process early. Her passion was about building the minds of people so they could be the best versions of themselves. My aunt now suffers from Wernicke-Korsakoff Syndrome, a combination of two of the disorders that cause dementia. One of the most difficult parts of her journey is that there is nothing I, or anyone else, can do to help her remember the people and stories that were such an important part of who she is. That hurts.

I realize now that I took time for granted. Even though I loved them all, I took those stories for granted. I took those memories for granted like they would always be there. I'm sure, at some point, there were things my aunt said that she would never forget, like her daughter. And now those memories are gone. The day that I heard my aunt call her daughter her sister, forever changed me. It broke my heart for one of the smartest people I have ever met. It broke my heart for my cousin because I can't imagine being in that situation. Except... I can... because my aunt/my godmother doesn't know who I am. So selfishly, my heart breaks for me as well.

As much as I want to say that I will never forget the times she and I shared... her tricking me into eating carrots and telling me they were sweet potatoes; working on my school science projects; her making me decide whether I was going to fight her or go back outside and fight bullies that ran me home; or simply reminiscing about all the family stories... The truth of the matter is, now that I know that African Americans are twice as likely to suffer from dementia as Caucasians, I'm not as confident that I will never forget her, others or even the stories I remember today. And that twice as likely statistic is projected to get worse over the next 15-20 years. But what I can say is that I will cherish every memory while I can, and I will cherish the people in my life while I can.

Tomorrow is not promised. What *is* promised is the present. And right now, I want to say I am thankful for every moment I have experienced with the people I love, and those who love me. I pray that I have made an impression on their lives like my aunt has made on mine. I will value the present even more than I ever have because I don't want to look back and regret not saying or doing something with them. I challenge you to do the same.

I am passionate about sharing this knowledge and these stories about dementia with you with hopes you and your loved ones will enjoy one another for a long time.

About the Author

C. Nathaniel Brown

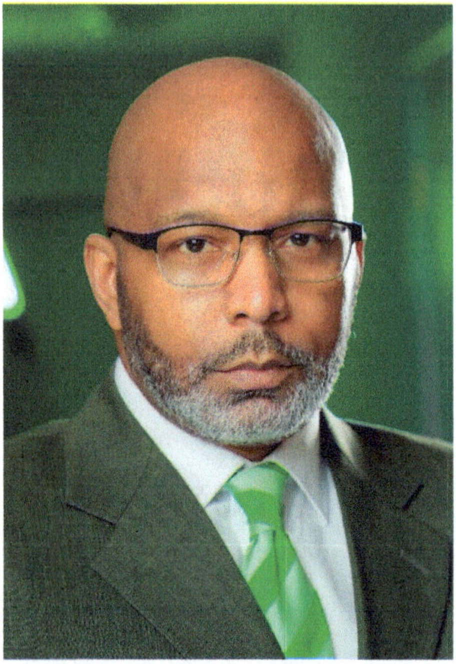

C. Nathaniel Brown is an award-winning writer, director, producer, and writing coach based in Atlanta, Georgia. Born and raised in Baltimore, Md., to a single mother, Chuck, as he is affectionately called, always dreamt of becoming a professional writer. After spending more than 20-plus years as a newspaper and magazine writer and editor, he opened a photography studio in Pittsburgh. In 2011, he moved to Atlanta to pursue his love for both the media and entertainment industries. He founded Expected End Entertainment LLC, a full-service media and entertainment company that focuses on creating content for the big screen, television, the internet, and books. Since establishing EX3, he has produced nearly 40 films, including feature films, documentaries and short films. He has also written more than 50 scripts. In addition, he is an author of 21 books and has helped thousands of writers become published authors and screenwriters. In his spare time, he enjoys eating pizza, watching movies, and spending time with family and friends. The father of two grown children and grandfather of four boys, he desires to impact the world by fulfilling the company's vision of Entertaining, Educating and Empowering others.

RESOURCES

FOR DEMENTIA PATIENTS

&

FOR CAREGIVERS

RESOURCES FOR PEOPLE WITH DEMENTIA

1. Alzheimer's Association: A leading organization offering resources, support groups, educational materials, and information about Alzheimer's and other dementias. Website: www.alz.org
2. Dementia Friends: An initiative that raises awareness and understanding of dementia, offering informative sessions to help individuals become more dementia-friendly. Website: www.dementiafriends.org
3. National Institute on Aging (NIA): Provides comprehensive information on aging-related topics, including dementia research, caregiving tips, and resources for individuals with dementia. Website: www.nia.nih.gov/alzheimers
4. AARP Caregiving Resource Center: Offers resources and support for caregivers, including articles, webinars, and tools for managing caregiving responsibilities. Website: www.aarp.org/caregiving
5. Family Caregiver Alliance: Provides caregiver resources, fact sheets, and online support groups for families dealing with dementia and other chronic illnesses. Website: www.caregiver.org
6. Dementia Care Central: Offers practical tips, resources, and information for caregivers of individuals with dementia. Website: www.dementiacarecentral.com
7. Lewy Body Dementia Association (LBDA): Focuses on raising awareness and providing support for individuals and families affected by Lewy body dementia. Website: www.lbda.org

8. Parkinson's Foundation: Offers resources and support for individuals with Parkinson's disease, which can sometimes lead to Parkinson's disease dementia. Website: www.parkinson.org
9. AgingCare: Provides articles, expert advice, and caregiver forums to help families navigate the challenges of caring for older adults with dementia. Website: www.agingcare.com
10. MemoryCare.com: Offers information about dementia types, care options, and resources to help families make informed decisions. Website: www.memorycare.com
11. National Alliance for Caregiving: Provides research, publications, and support for caregivers dealing with dementia and other chronic conditions. Website: www.caregiving.org
12. CaringBridge: Allows caregivers to create a private online journal to update family and friends on a loved one's dementia journey. Website: www.caringbridge.org
13. MindMate: Offers an app with cognitive exercises, brain-training games, and tools to support memory and cognitive function. Website: www.mindmate-app.com
14. The Dementia Society: Provides educational resources, caregiver support, and workshops for families affected by dementia. Website: www.dementiasociety.org
15. National Stroke Association: Offers resources for individuals dealing with vascular dementia, which can result from strokes. Website: www.stroke.org

16. Medicare: Provides information about Medicare coverage for dementia-related services, medications, and care. Website: www.medicare.gov
17. Alzheimer's Research UK: Offers resources on dementia research, understanding different forms of dementia, and ways to get involved. Website: www.alzheimersresearchuk.org
18. The Caregiver Space: An online community where caregivers can connect, share stories, and find support from others in similar situations. Website: www.thecaregiverspace.org
19. Eldercare Locator: A resource from the U.S. Administration on Aging that helps individuals find local support services for older adults and caregivers. Website: www.eldercare.acl.gov
20. Aging in Place: Offers tips, resources, and guidance for creating a safe and comfortable environment for individuals with dementia to age in place. Website: www.aginginplace.org
21. Being Patient: Provides articles, videos, and personal stories about living with dementia, caregiving, and the latest dementia research. Website: www.beingpatient.com
22. Caregiver Action Network: Offers practical tips, educational resources, and support for caregivers of individuals with dementia and other health conditions. Website: www.caregiveraction.org
23. Alzheimer's Foundation of America: Provides resources, educational materials, and a helpline for individuals and

families affected by dementia. Website: www.alzfdn.org

24. Dementia Friends USA: Offers information and resources to raise awareness and understanding of dementia in communities across the United States. Website: www.dementiafriendsusa.org
25. Dementia Society of America: Provides education, advocacy, and support for individuals and families affected by various forms of dementia. Website: www.dementiasociety.org
26. ARCH National Respite Network and Resource Center: Offers information about respite care options for caregivers needing temporary relief. Website: www.archrespite.org
27. American Association for Geriatric Psychiatry: Provides resources and information about mental health and dementia in older adults. Website: www.aagponline.org
28. CurePSP: Offers resources and support for individuals and families dealing with progressive supranuclear palsy (PSP) and related disorders. Website: www.psp.org
29. Dementia Australia: Provides information, support, and resources for individuals with dementia and their caregivers in Australia. Website: www.dementia.org.au
30. Well Spouse Association: Offers support, resources, and a community for spouses and partners caring for loved ones with chronic illnesses, including dementia. Website: www.wellspouse.org
31. Alter: Alter equips faith communities with practical tools and resources needed to support their members

living with dementia and their caregivers. Website: www.AlterDementia.com

32. The Association for Frontotemporal Denegeration (AFTD): AFTD's mission is to improve the quality of life of people affected by FTD and drive research to a cure. Website: www.theAFTD.org

RESOURCES FOR CAREGIVERS

1. Alzheimer's Association Caregiver Center: Offers caregiver resources, support groups, tips, and information about caring for individuals with Alzheimer's and other dementias. Website: www.alz.org/care
2. Family Caregiver Alliance: Provides a wealth of resources, including caregiver support groups, fact sheets, and online tools for caregivers dealing with dementia and other chronic illnesses. Website: www.caregiver.org
3. ARCH National Respite Network and Resource Center: Offers information about respite care options for caregivers needing temporary relief from their caregiving responsibilities. Website: www.archrespite.org
4. AARP Caregiving Resource Center: Provides articles, webinars, and tools to help caregivers manage their caregiving roles and responsibilities. Website: www.aarp.org/caregiving
5. Caregiver Action Network: Offers resources, tips, and educational materials for caregivers dealing with dementia and other health conditions. Website: www.caregiveraction.org
6. Caring.com: Offers a range of articles, forums, and resources for caregivers, including those caring for individuals with dementia. Website: www.caring.com
7. Eldercare Locator: A resource from the U.S. Administration on Aging that helps caregivers find local

support services for older adults, including those with dementia. Website: www.eldercare.acl.gov

8. Well Spouse Association: Provides support, resources, and a community for spouses and partners caring for loved ones with chronic illnesses, including dementia. Website: www.wellspouse.org
9. National Alliance for Caregiving: Offers research, publications, and support for caregivers dealing with dementia and other chronic conditions. Website: www.caregiving.org
10. AgingCare: Provides articles, expert advice, and caregiver forums to help caregivers navigate the challenges of caring for older adults with dementia. Website: www.agingcare.com
11. Alzheimer's Foundation of America: Offers resources, educational materials, and a helpline for caregivers of individuals with Alzheimer's and other dementias. Website: www.alzfdn.org
12. Caregiver Space: An online community where caregivers can connect, share stories, and find support from others in similar caregiving situations. Website: www.thecaregiverspace.org
13. CurePSP: Offers resources and support for caregivers dealing with progressive supranuclear palsy (PSP) and related disorders. Website: www.psp.org
14. ARCH Caregiver Materials: Provides resources and materials specifically designed to support caregivers of individuals with dementia. Website: www.archrespite.org/caregivers

15. Lotsa Helping Hands: Offers a platform for caregivers to coordinate support from family, friends, and volunteers in caregiving tasks. Website: www.lotsahelpinghands.com
16. Caregiver Support Services: Provides online courses, workshops, and resources to empower caregivers with knowledge and skills. Website: www.caregiversupportservices.com
17. DailyCaring: Offers practical tips, advice, and resources for caregivers of individuals with dementia to make caregiving tasks more manageable. Website: www.dailycaring.com
18. Aging in Place: Offers tips, resources, and guidance for caregivers to create a safe and comfortable environment for individuals with dementia to age in place. Website: www.aginginplace.org
19. Alzheimer's Society (UK): Offers caregiver support, resources, and information for those caring for individuals with dementia in the United Kingdom. Website: www.alzheimers.org.uk
20. Age UK: Provides resources, advice, and support for caregivers of older adults, including those with dementia, in the United Kingdom. Website: www.ageuk.org.uk
21. Dementia Society of America: Offers education, advocacy, and support for caregivers dealing with various forms of dementia. Website: www.dementiasociety.org
22. Carers UK: Provides resources, support, and information for caregivers in the United Kingdom,

including those caring for individuals with dementia. Website: www.carersuk.org

23. Aging and Disability Resource Centers (ADRCs): Offers information, resources, and assistance for caregivers seeking support services for older adults with dementia. Website: Search for ADRCs in your location.
24. HelpGuide: Provides articles and resources on dementia caregiving, including self-care tips for caregivers. Website: www.helpguide.org
25. Medicare: Offers information about Medicare coverage for dementia-related services, caregiving support, and resources. Website: www.medicare.gov
26. Dementia Friends USA: Offers resources to raise awareness and understanding of dementia, supporting caregivers and promoting dementia-friendly communities. Website: www.dementiafriendsusa.org
27. National Caregivers Library: Provides a wide range of resources, articles, and checklists to support caregivers in their caregiving roles. Website: www.caregiverslibrary.org
28. The Rosalynn Carter Institute for Caregiving: Offers resources, training, and support for caregivers to enhance their caregiving skills and well-being. Website: www.rosalynncarter.org
29. Wellness Works: Provides resources, workshops, and tools to promote self-care and well-being for caregivers of individuals with dementia. Website: www.wellnessworksmp.com
30. Being Patient: Offers articles, videos, and personal stories about caregiving for individuals with dementia,

as well as the latest dementia research. Website: www.beingpatient.com

31. Georgia Department of Human Services Division of Aging Services: The department crafted a plan to address Alzheimer's and related dementia called Georgia Alzheimer's & Related Dementias State Plan. Website: https://aging.georgia.gov/get-involved/georgia-alzheimers-related-dementias-state-plan
32. Senior 911: A Georgia-based company that provides senior home care for clients with dementia. Website: www.Senior911.org
33. Second Wind Dreams: The organization hosts virtual dementia tours and other educational programs around dementia. Website: https://www.secondwind.org/
34. Deluxe Senior Care: An Atlanta, Georgia company that provides personalized in-home senior care services, specializing in care for dementia patients. Website: www.deluxeseniorcare.com